For further copies of this booklet
Email: info@youcanhelp.com.au

ACKNOWLEDGMENTS

Reviewers (back cover):

Dr Mark Wenitong
Adjunct Associate Professor, James Cook University, School of Tropical Public Health,
Aboriginal Public Health Medical Officer at NACCHO,
Senior Medical Advisor at Apunipima Cape York Health Council

Professor John Macdonald
Foundation Chair in Primary Health Care, Director,
Men's Health Information and Resource Centre, Western Sydney University

HEALTH SERVICE AND PRACTITIONER REVIEWERS

Angela Dufek
Senior Manager: Client Services,
Port Lincoln Aboriginal Health Service, South Australia

George Laslett
Drug and Alcohol Services Manager,
Umoona Tjutagku Health Service Aboriginal Corporation, Coober Pedy

Roger Fielke
Senior Mental Health Nurse,
(Locum in East Arnhem Land Northern Territory)

Anthony Smith
Consultant Educator (male mental health and suicide prevention),
Australian Institute of Male Health and Studies

GRAPHIC DESIGN Green Pigeon Graphics – Johanna Evans

GENERAL EDITING Cynthia Collins

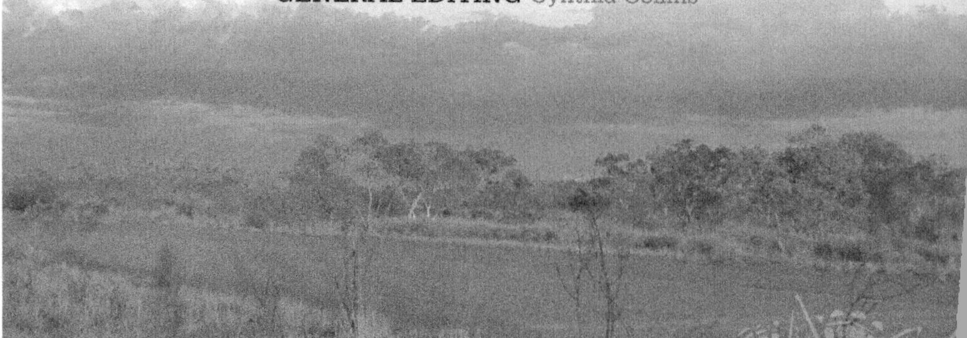

Preventing Suicide in Indigenous Communities

Essential reading for those who aim to make a difference

Contents

The Purpose of this Resource

Preventing Suicide in Indigenous Communities aims to build the knowledge capacity of social and emotional wellbeing workers, community leaders, health and mental health workers and key community members. It is the product of experience working in suicide prevention and mental health in a number of Indigenous communities and consideration of literature and reports published by Indigenous Elders, academics, NGO and government sources. It has also depended on the kind assistance of several reviewers associated with Indigenous health and community organisations.

It is not intended to be a 'one size fits all' resource. It is beyond the scope of such a resource to reflect the culture, social history, conditions or needs of each indigenous community. Nor can it cater for people who are non-literate in English and who might benefit from a resource in their own language. Instead it sets out to inform Indigenous and non-indigenous people in key roles in communities – people who are English literate and have active links to community services, institutions and organisations. These people are often the ones who can make things happen and are best placed to know the cultural and social characteristics and needs of the communities in which they live.

Though this resource is relevant to both male and female suicide prevention, it is important to recognise that the majority of Aboriginal and Torres Strait Islander suicides are male – young males. It is remarkable that, though most suicides are male, little effort has gone into understanding the particular experience and psychology of males in current suicide prevention efforts. Nor is this yet generally a consideration of researchers, program developers and funding bodies. This should not be taken to suggest that we understand the gender specific experience and needs of females at risk of suicide; in fact, a lack of gender specific understanding in relation to females at risk of suicide is also problematic for prevention efforts.

Obviously, the information in a resource of this kind – in fact the sum of literature on this subject, is no substitute for strong culture, changed social conditions, or the need for more relevant programs and services in Aboriginal and Torres Strait Islander communities. However, practical and accessible information is needed, to help empower key people, who are in a position to influence programs, services and community thinking and action, with relevant 'rules of thumb' and useful ideas.

A section on *Teenagers and Self-harm* has been included, because of the frequency of self-harm in Indigenous communities, the importance of understanding the different approaches that are needed in response to self-harm compared with suicidal thinking and behaviour and because, though self-harm is most often not suicidal behaviour, repeated self-harm makes suicide potentially a less foreign and statistically more likely one.

For the sake of brevity, Aboriginal and Torres Strait Islander people will be referred to throughout this resource as Indigenous people.

The tragedy and challenge of Indigenous suicide

"Death is our life," said an Aboriginal elder from South Australia, describing the tragic experience of many Aboriginal communities Australia-wide, of mourning and sadness for too many young lives lost.

There are simply no words to adequately describe the depth of grief and pain felt by families and communities due to suicide. Unlike death due to sickness, old age, or even accident, suicide creates unanswerable questions that plague the mind and gives rise to emotions of regret, anguish and powerlessness that burn like acid. The aftermath of suicide is human misery of the worst kind. With each suicide the fabric of family and community is torn, their capacity for resilience is damaged and their health and wellbeing compromised.

Suicide prevention should be one of the most urgent priorities of our times – especially in Aboriginal and Torres Strait Islander communities.

A plentiful number of published reports, strategic models, recommendations and research findings are available, yet these are too often not followed by action. Still the rate of suicide remains stubbornly and tragically high. Prevention of suicide in Indigenous communities by outside government agencies and programs – especially those with a mental illness focus, have made small if any gains. Suicide is a national disgrace and one that belies our assertions of the value of human life and community.

Indigenous people who know and see their communities from the 'inside' have repeatedly asserted the need for a *community centred approach*, one that harnesses cultural resources – including elders and key community leaders of culture, in order to begin to heal the wounds of the past and the loss of self-identity and to find confidence and strength to face and overcome the challenges of the future.

The aftermath of suicide is human misery of the worst kind. With each suicide the fabric of family and community is torn, their capacity for resilience is damaged and their health and wellbeing compromised.

In support of healthy culture is the need to urgently address the many adverse social conditions and circumstances of indigenous communities. Any initiatives must be sensitive to local communities and arising from them. Outside resources will of course be crucial, but they will be most effective if they support initiatives of local origin and ownership: creative and flexible ways of doing things that reach beyond the imagination and scope of uniform and generalised bureaucratic policies and programs.

Outside resources will of course be crucial, but they will be most effective if they support initiatives of local origin and ownership: creative and flexible ways of doing things that reach beyond the imagination and scope of uniform and generalised bureaucratic policies and programs.

Too many lives lost – the facts

- Suicide is one of the most common causes of death among Aboriginal and Torres Strait Islander peoples.
- Suicide accounts for 1 in 20 Indigenous deaths and with the problem of under-reporting this rate is very likely higher.
- Nearly 80% of all suicides in Australia are male, with two thirds dying on their first attempt.
- Males are around 3.3 times more likely to die by suicide than females.
- Young Aboriginal and Torres Strait Islander males (15-19 years) are over 4 times more likely to die by suicide than are other young Australian males. Similarly, young Aboriginal and Torres Strait Islander females (15-19 years) are nearly 6 times more likely to die by suicide than are other young females. These rates of suicide are amongst the highest in the world.
- Self-harm is common in Indigenous communities, particularly amongst adolescents. Individuals who self-harm are up to 200 times at greater risk of suicide than the general population across the lifespan.
- Of great concern is how suicide deaths often spark clusters of suicides (suicide contagion) in Indigenous communities.
- Most disturbing is that increasingly children are committing suicide and may be perceiving suicide as an almost normal behaviour; that some children are beginning to see ending their lives as the only available coping mechanism signals serious community breakdown.
- Suicide rates in rural and remote areas are significantly greater than in urban populations, with indigenous males being most at risk.
- Alcohol intoxication hugely increases the risk of suicide and the impulsiveness that is often associated with it.
- Current emphases of services offering intervention with mental illness do not appear to be successful in suicide prevention in Indigenous communities.
- Depression and suicide are sometimes linked. However, this link should not automatically be assumed, because there are many cases where no such link is evident. Automatically assuming this link can also obscure other factors influencing suicide, such as psychological distress and powerlessness.

- Current evidence does not support the idea that antidepressants are useful in reducing the risk of suicide attempts or completions. They may in fact have potential to heighten the risk of suicide across all age groups.
- Families of Aboriginal children have reported extraordinarily high levels of stress.

  In one survey, findings suggested that 1 in 5 Aboriginal children aged 0-17 years experienced living in families where major life stress events – incarceration, violence, severe hardship and death – had occurred.
- Suicide deaths, particularly by hanging, have frequently been witnessed by members of Indigenous communities and places where people have died by suicide have often taken on local meanings and associations. There are examples of communities with high levels of exposure to both death and suicide that appear to have become desensitised to suicide and self-harm, so that these behaviours, though not acceptable, have become 'normal' and even expected.

Communities, families and individuals most at risk of suicide

Suicide in Indigenous communities not only appears associated with conditions and factors in common with non-indigenous people who end their lives, but must also be understood in the context of a whole extra layer of complex underlying historical, social, cultural and economic problems and conditions – which have been found to greatly contribute to increased individual risk and endemic rates of suicide and self-harm among Indigenous peoples.

It would be misleading to suggest a list of definitive risk factors relating to community, family, or individuals, given this complexity. Some risk factors in current literature are not yet strongly supported with data, though corroborated by communities' own observations and those of workers and health professionals in Indigenous communities. Also, only limited research has been conducted into Indigenous understandings and definitions of suicide and self-harm behaviour.

More knowledge derived from research and evaluation of existing programs of prevention will

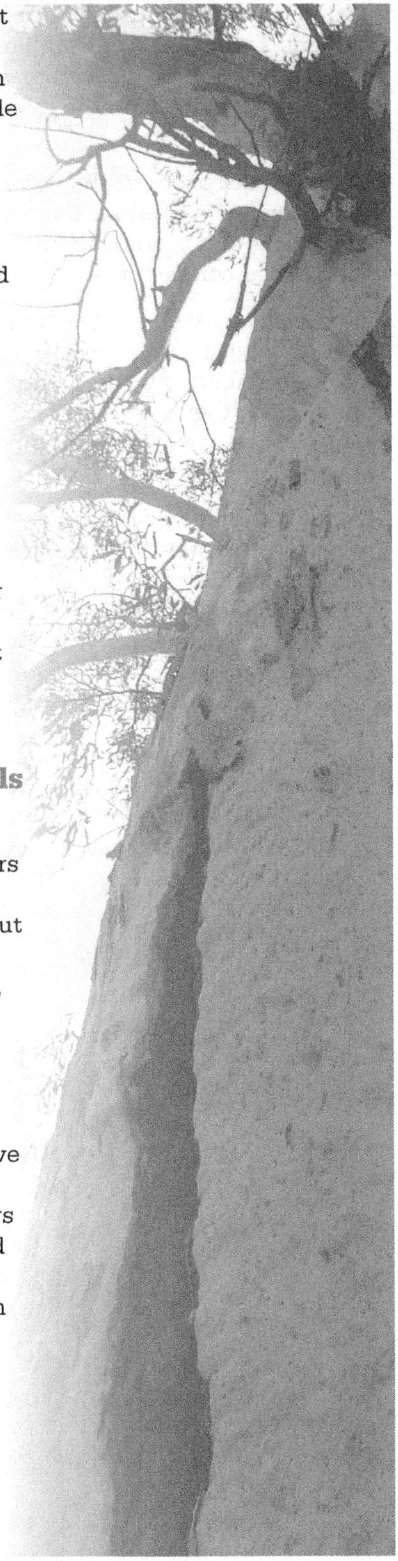

need to continue to inform our efforts and thus bring us closer to more effective solutions. Despite the present limitations of suicide prevention knowledge, enough is known to act with reasonable confidence in attempting to make real headway in diminishing the rates of suicide in both indigenous and non-indigenous communities.

And let us not overlook the potential merit of finding out what does appear to be working in some contexts and more fully resourcing those efforts – doing more of what works and tentatively replicating those features that may be generalisable for other similar communities.

The health and wellbeing of Indigenous peoples is not an insoluble problem, especially if capacity for prevention can be nurtured within communities by communities themselves and if they can find ways of engaging – especially young people, with the transformative power of culture.

Given the formidable challenges and pressures facing Indigenous communities, families and individuals, one can only marvel at the strength and resilience of Indigenous peoples, when so many families have still been able to raise healthy, happy children and maintain and nurture their culture in many regions of Australia.

The health and wellbeing of Indigenous peoples is not an insoluble problem, especially if capacity for prevention can be nurtured within communities by communities themselves and if they can find ways of engaging – especially young people, with the transformative power of culture.

Community risk factors that may heighten the likelihood of suicide

- Bereavement and grief overload due to too many deaths from various causes
- Detrimental effects of intergenerational transmission of grief and trauma
- Significant sense of powerlessness
- Anger and rage emanating from a sense of powerlessness
- Felt sense of having been dispossessed, displaced and marginalised
- Conflicting sense of being 'caught between two cultures'
- Poverty – including continuing subsistence income, lack of access to information, essential services, good nutrition and opportunities for improvement
- Over-familiarity with death for indigenous children
- Self-harm having become a common behaviour of young people and being observed by children in the community
- Unemployment, underemployment and lack of meaningful employment
- Lack of appropriate housing and overcrowding
- Widespread use of illicit and harmful drugs
- Mental health difficulties are not identified, and individuals experiencing psychological distress are not adequately supported
- Heavy drinking – high risk use of alcohol
- Loss of cultural connections and identity
- Separation of children from parents and child removal by government authorities
- A high incidence of child protection orders and out of home care
- Experience of and matters arising out of family law: such as child removal, custody disputes, relationship conflict, child access and support arrangements and interfamily enmity
- High levels of psychological distress

- Suicides in the community with the potential to give rise to a cluster effect, or suicide contagion
- Strong community feeling of alienation
- Fractured community and family links and conflictual relationships
- Negative impact of unhelpful government policies and programs
- Poor status and demonization and marginalisation of males in the community
- Poor English literacy – making it difficult to navigate government information, services and bureaucratic requirements and poor or deteriorating literacy in traditional languages, making it difficult to maintain the health and integrity of traditional culture
- Disputes and conflict between local and recently arrived community members of different Indigenous origins (of country) over jobs, local leadership and accepted local cultural norms
- Not enough publicly recognised leaders, role models and mentors
- Weakened role of local elders
- Breakdown in community support of families
- Child abuse and neglect
- Welfare dependence
- Health and welfare services that operate outside communities and that do not effectively consult, connect with and adapt to community needs
- Government and NGO programs that are short-lived and not sustainable due to funding arrangements and changes in government and government policy (personnel also often change too frequently for relationships to be built with key people and communities)
- Overt and covert racism experienced from the wider non-indigenous community and institutional racism inherent in past and present government policies affecting Indigenous communities
- Sexual assault
- Family violence
- Violence as an increasingly normative and taken for granted behaviour in the community (payback, is a cultural practice now often practised out of frustration and alcohol or substance fuelled)
- High levels of psychological distress in the community

Responding to Community risk factors:

Need for a cross sector and multidisciplinary approach

Indigenous suicide is most commonly defined as a mental health issue (the domain of mental health services), with some prevention efforts being addressed by other non-mental health services. Whilst better mental health services for Indigenous communities are needed, this approach tends to conflate suicide with mental illness – especially depression. This has been found to contribute little to suicide prevention, and is misleading, since suicide is mostly attributable to psychological distress and situational factors not mental disorder or illness.

More effective prevention will be achieved by equipping human service oriented non-mental illness focused service providers, disciplines, and sectors with better knowledge of preventative strategies and messaging, in carrying out a primary prevention role and in addressing situational factors. Much needed is an approach that tackles social determinants, the vulnerabilities of communities, and that supports community initiatives aimed at families and individuals experiencing psychological distress.

Building community capacity

Communities need to be helped to develop the capacity to take care of themselves. Key individuals need to be trained in community development principles and in how to prioritise and address high risk factors for suicide in Indigenous communities.

Community capacity building for preventative mental health and suicide prevention is essential. Waiting for people at risk to turn up at mental health clinics or outreach services has contributed little to suicide prevention and in fact largely misses the point. Crisis interventions are important when needed, but do nothing to address the community and social conditions giving rise to suicide

Key individuals also need to be trained to conduct basic community education in preventative mental health and suicide prevention. Their task will be concerned with finding ways of strengthening community mental health and wellbeing and endeavouring to prevent people from getting to the point of needing mental health crisis interventions.

It is also high time we revisited and demystified the whole notion of mental health, avoiding unnecessary labels of 'disorder' and 'illness' (which serve only to pathologise individuals), and making it no longer the preserve of mental health services and professionals, instead rendering preventative mental health and suicide prevention an empowering capacity of individuals and their communities.

More appropriate mental health services and collaboration

Appropriately oriented mental health services are much needed to support Indigenous communities; however, they need to engage much more directly with these communities by reaching out to them and getting to know families and individuals in their everyday context of living. Community leaders have posed the question: "how can you know who is hurting in our community if you are sitting in an office?"

Mental health services need to focus much more on high prevalence mental health difficulties and early intervention models of service delivery, rather than waiting for people with minor or developing problems to later find themselves in mental health crisis. Acute mental health services will continue to be overwhelmed as long as too little effort of promotion, prevention and early intervention for mental health is occurring. There needs to be the leadership and resolve to change service orientation. Such a change will not only win the support of communities (who will feel more like service providers care about them) but will result in improved economy: a better utilisation of scarce resources.

Acute mental health services will continue to be overwhelmed as long as little effort of promotion, prevention and early intervention for mental health is occurring.

Integration of services is also important. Community liaison workers, social and emotional wellbeing workers (common in Indigenous health services), can play a crucial role in preventative mental health and suicide prevention by working in close collaboration with counsellors, psychologists, mental health practitioners, community nurses and GPs in providing a seamless and comprehensive support for the mental health of Indigenous communities. This does not require endless time wasting meetings, but merely some clear terms of reference, professional and effective communication and information sharing, out of respect and concern for what is in the best interests of clients (the Port Lincoln Aboriginal Health Service is a notable example of a health service that has initiated this model).

An untapped potential resource is videoconferencing, which could be used to offer high quality psychology, psychotherapy, and counselling services that simply cannot be located or are not feasible to locate in some communities. As band width problems are resolved particularly in rural and remote communities by extension of the NBN, a whole new range of services can be offered. This can be done using fixed unit hardware or portable devices like tablets. This technology has been trialled and has been successful in rural and outback communities. It can also be used to provide static and audio-visual information – as an alternative to some printed health promotion materials. With the easy addition of touch screen capacity, it can be used to simplify the interface between people of poor English literacy and the administrative requirements of city bureaucracies with whom Indigenous people sometimes have to deal. Much depends on appropriately tailored software and properly designed system specifications and support.

Grief and after suicide support of communities

Appropriate responses to the enduring grief experienced within Indigenous communities as a result of suicide needs to be addressed as a matter of priority as part of all Indigenous suicide prevention efforts. Providing grief and after suicide support should include a whole-of-community approach which fosters dialogue and awareness of the need for vigilance, particularly around young people, as a strategy for reducing cluster suicides. Indigenous and non-Indigenous workers and service providers need to be appropriately trained to respond proactively and sensitively to suicide deaths and suicide attempts occurring within Indigenous communities.

Opportunities for housing and work

Two of the most important determinants of family and community health and wellbeing, are whether or not people have an appropriate place to live and meaningful remunerative work. Overcrowding and unemployment are key markers of poverty – poverty that breeds misery, social decline and many of the risk factors of suicide. When these issues are addressed in communities, startling outcomes can occur and many other social and family issues begin to resolve.

When these issues are addressed in communities, startling outcomes can occur and many other social and family issues begin to resolve.

Mental health promotion and efforts of suicide prevention cannot succeed in environments where these basic needs are not met.

Men especially, need to work to maintain their mental health and psychological wellbeing. Men, much more than women, tend to define themselves and are defined by their community – and given status, according to their productive capacity through work. Living on welfare is demeaning and all too commonly leads to a decline in physical and mental health. Welfare dependence should be considered a risk factor contributing to the overall risk of suicide for Indigenous communities. The erosion of culture and men's roles in particular by welfare or 'sit down money' should not be underestimated. Men need to work and any suicide prevention strategy that doesn't take this into account will be deficient.

Managing alcohol and substances in communities

Many Indigenous communities are ravaged by alcohol and substance misuse. This will continue to fuel family violence, foetal alcohol syndrome, poor mental health, dementia and suicide, unless it is better managed.

In some communities this misuse – particularly bingeing, is exacerbated by a cultural and historical survival practice of 'feast or famine' – that of quickly consuming and sharing what is available until it is fully used. In some communities where alcohol is controlled, a strong smuggling trade with lucrative profits has also developed, creating even greater challenges for programs of community care.

Again, these problems cannot be tackled effectively without at the same time addressing other social and community factors and conditions, such as overcrowding, unemployment and poverty.

The role of local leadership will be crucial in offering an example to others of appropriate alcohol use. In making a transition to the more appropriate use of alcohol, communities will need ready access to detoxification, medical and community support services. Such services will also be needed to cope with the increasing use of substances in many Indigenous communities. Much may be gained by closer cooperation between community leaders, locally available drug and alcohol workers and police. In the case of both alcohol and substance abuse, education beginning with schools may play a vitally important preventative role.

The role of local leadership will be crucial in offering an example to others of appropriate alcohol use.

Engaging youth

With young people being most at risk of suicide in Indigenous communities, creative strategies for their engagement in the life of their communities, their culture and in acquiring important life skills and competencies are much needed. They will need to be engaged in a range of settings including at school, in the community, in the workplace and through participation in sports and the arts. Peer leadership and peer support training, the use of mentors and engagement with Elders of the community and especially programs like the award-winning *Yirimam Project* and its intergenerational 'on country' program, may be of great benefit.

More effective approach to family violence

Recent publicity about family violence in Australian is doing much to highlight a problem in urgent need of understanding and action.

Indigenous families and communities, women, children and men, need to feel safe from violence, but if that is to happen a quite different, more broadly and accurately informed approach will be needed. Most immediately, leaders in communities, both men and women, can become part of the solution by setting up mechanisms to ensure safety to anyone who feels threatened with any form of violence and by commencing community conversations about the issue of domestic and other forms of violence and what can be done practically to bring about change.

Taking young people onto country – especially traditional land, is considered a strong basis for building self-belief, self-identity, self-confidence and self-respect.

Strengthening culture and cultural connections

There is evidence to suggest that strengthening connections with traditional Indigenous culture and the land may be a significant protective factor in suicide prevention. Indigenous communities themselves have repeatedly emphasised that these connections are vital in addressing the vulnerability of young people to suicide and self-harm. Taking young people onto country – especially traditional land, is considered a strong basis for building self-belief, self-identity, self-confidence and self-respect. In a rapidly changing world, going out bush becomes even more important as a way of practicing culture, reinforcing cultural identity and as one

Elder put it: "learning who we are again". And, "what better way to find out what is happening for at-risk teenagers than taking them out fishing, hunting, or just sitting down with them on country?"

More attention needs to be paid to Indigenous males

In Australia, suicide is now the number one killer of men under 44 years of age. And though by far the majority of suicides are male, little attention is given to suicide as a predominantly male behaviour and a behaviour that can only be understood from the gender specific perspective of male experience and male psychology; in the case of Indigenous males, their own particular circumstances, experience, cultural background and orientation.

Because Indigenous male suicides play an important part in explaining elevated suicide rates in Indigenous communities, with many suicides concentrated in the 15 to 24 and 25 to 34 age brackets, much more attention needs to be paid to the experience and struggles of Indigenous males.

Because Indigenous male suicides play an important part in explaining elevated suicide rates in Indigenous communities, with many suicides concentrated in the 15 to 24 and 25 to 34 age brackets, much more attention needs to be paid to the experience and struggles of Indigenous males.

It should come as no surprise that we have seen little progress in the health and mental health status of Indigenous males and their communities. Endeavours to improve community health status and community development driven by Indigenous women are commendable and of vital importance. These women have often 'risen to the occasion' in support of their menfolk and children. For some men though, this trend has led to an increased sense of failure, shame and despair. Without the engagement of Aboriginal men, not only will males very likely remain at much higher risk of suicide, but the progress of communities towards better health and wellbeing in general will be severely limited. In many communities men are not significantly engaged in community life and are being left behind. Many Indigenous men experience powerlessness, social disenfranchisement and alienation and too often feel like they live on the margins of their own communities.

Only if Indigenous manhood is reinstated and if Indigenous men are encouraged to rediscover pride in their gender identity, in themselves, in their culture and in roles central to community life, will communities be able to engage creatively with the problems and challenges that face them and anticipate the future with optimism.

Careful thought needs to go into developing men's groups and activities that can not only begin a process of reclaiming men for their communities, but that can also serve as a place for younger males to be mentored and supported with all the demands of their growing up to be men.

Peer support training, such as *Menswatch*, has proved highly successful with groups of Indigenous men. Using all-male groups, it trains men to be a key resource in their communities, to be aware of and to respond to the distress of other men and to provide support, or when professional help is needed, referral to an appropriate service, or health professional. It combines training in preventative mental health, suicide prevention, helping skills, risk assessment and some of the basics of male psychology.

Only if Indigenous manhood is reinstated and if Indigenous men are encouraged to rediscover pride in their gender identity, in themselves, in their culture and in roles central to community life, will communities be able to engage creatively with the problems and challenges that face them and anticipate the future with optimism.

A lost generation of boys

The tragic loss of life of young Indigenous males yells from the suicide data as a priority issue. And yet little attention is given to this in suicide research and prevention efforts. Whatever stands in the way of gender specific consideration of suicide, it's time we counted the cost of allowing such an impediment to continue.

With so much emphasis in our society generally on child health and welfare, childhood development, child rearing, parenting and education, it seems extraordinary that, when it comes to the profoundly consequential matter of transition from childhood to adulthood, the young are left largely unsupported; they are, in effect, left to their own devices. The problem, of course, is that their own devices originate from their own immaturity and are not informed by the wisdom or attributes of mature adulthood.

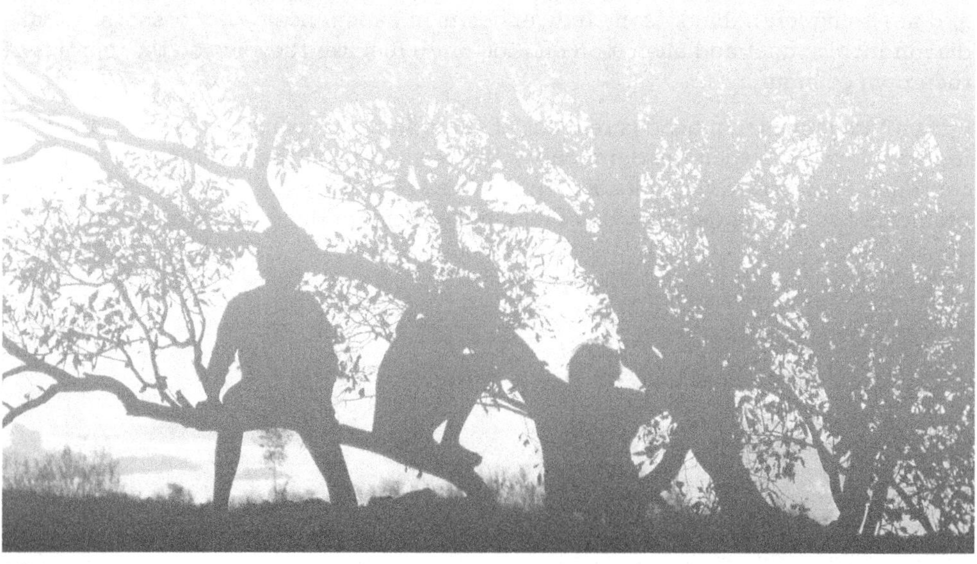

Young males left without assistance in this transition, frequently resort to means that are dangerous and often harmful to themselves and sometimes to others. Their desperate yet misguided bid to prove themselves worthy of inclusion in the adult world of men is expressed through the abuse of alcohol, through many forms of dangerous risk taking, through violence, aggression, destructiveness, trophy-sex, public posturing and by using and abusing others. Such attempts at 'self-initiation' usually merely result in a more toughened, strident and aggressive version of *boy psychology*.

Young males left without assistance in this transition, frequently resort to means that are dangerous and often harmful to themselves and sometimes to others.

The difficulty of this transition is greatly amplified for young Indigenous males who are without role models, mentors, or the functional role of male elders. It can only add to the level of suicide risk – risk potently conspicuous in male youth suicide statistics.

The problem of unsupported and consequently unsuccessful transition from *boy psychology* to *man psychology* is obviously not just one experienced at the time of manhood-aspiring adolescence; it is carried into and throughout male adult life.

Many men remain boys, failing to progress to mature manhood, not because they want to, but because no one has shown them how.

Young males need proper processes and means for making a supported transition from boyhood to mature manhood. Only a community of men – mature men who have come to grips with their own issues of self-identity, can provide the best context for this to happen. Such a community of men is absent in most communities because of many adverse social and historical factors. Nevertheless, it can and must be rebuilt if health is to be restored to communities and if pointless suicide deaths are to be avoided.

Young males need proper processes and means for making a supported transition from boyhood to mature manhood.

Self-determination and self-management

There is little doubt that communities which are properly supported to be self-determining and self-managing, when it comes to health and welfare service delivery and community development, generally have improved outcomes and declining suicide rates.

In communities where people have been diminished by poor health, poverty and entrenched social problems, self-determination requires resources to be put into leadership training and empowerment initiatives in parallel with concerted efforts to improve social and health conditions. It is also essential that Indigenous people have the opportunity to acquire training and qualifications in all fields pertaining to the roles they can play in bringing health, mental health, safety and wellbeing to their communities.

More targeted and locally informed printed resources and materials

Assistance with the development of targeted local printed resources and materials, informed by local culture, local insights and knowledge, will also be needed to support the efforts of communities in capacity building, health promotion and suicide prevention. Creative ways of using picture narratives and local languages have potential to be much more effective than the 'one size fits all' resources most often offered to communities for distribution to local people. Financial resources of some large Australian mental health promotion organisations – those that are funded by government and donor sources, could easily be used to achieve this with communities – especially given the urgency of addressing suicide amongst Indigenous peoples. Here again, preventative mental health needs to undergo reorientation in order to recognise not just individual risk factors, but also social determinants of suicide and deteriorating mental health.

Family risk factors that may heighten the likelihood of suicide

- Lack of meaningful wider family and community support networks
- Bereavement and grief overload due to too many deaths in the family or community
- Separation of children from parents, child removal or a child protection order initiated by government authorities
- Experience of and matters arising out of family law: such as child removal, custody disputes, relationship conflict, child access and support arrangements
- Involvement in or subject to interfamily enmity and conflict
- High levels of psychological distress in the family
- Having to travel significant distances away from home and bearing the burden and expense of accessing medical, court and other essential or mandatory appointments
- Supporting a family member with a mental health difficulty or physical disability
- Incarceration or return from incarceration of a parent or adolescent
- Child abuse or neglect in the family
- Welfare dependence
- Poor health (such as a chronic health condition) of family member(s)
- Poverty – including lack of access to information, essential services, good nutrition and opportunities for improvement
- Over-exposure of children in the family to death in the community
- Self-harm and risk taking behaviour – especially by adolescents
- Unemployment, underemployment, or lack of meaningful employment for adults in the family
- Overcrowding – too many people living in one house
- Use of illicit and harmful drugs by family member(s)

- A family member with a mental health difficulty that is not being adequately addressed
- Heavy drinking – high risk use of alcohol by family member(s)
- Family, intimate partner, sibling or elder violence
- Fear of reprisals and violence in inter-family disputes and conflict
- Fear of community violence; for the safety of children
- Overt and covert racism experienced from the wider non-indigenous community
- Males in the family feeling marginalised, alienated and angry
- Poor English literacy – making it difficult to navigate government information, services and bureaucratic requirements

Responding to Family risk factors:

Child training for later life

Since suicide risk is associated with adversity in early childhood, there is much to be gained by concentrating effort into early childhood development, health and education. Child and family services, schools and health services are in a powerful position to help build strengths, competencies and resilience in children, to protect them against sources of risk and adversity that make them vulnerable to self-harm in later life. Specific tailored program emphases or careful adaptations of relevant existing programs should be developed to address the challenges facing children in individual Indigenous communities.

Parenting skills training

There are no perfect parents and all parents can benefit from the shared pool of knowledge and skills that now exist for parenting more effectively. All the more needful are these in families that are beset by the complex difficulties and challenges of struggling communities.

Effective parenting can nurture vital resilience in children by cultivating personal and mutual respect, skills of conflict management, ability to manage emotions and to problem solve and by modelling appropriate help seeking. But parenting skills training will always be strengthened by the wisdom of older people in communities and needs to be accompanied by proper ongoing support for and valuing of parents themselves. It is important to have programs that are child focused, but unless parents are properly supported and valued small benefits occur.

Access to appropriate housing and good nutrition

The health and wellbeing of families depends in no small way on their ability to manage simple day-to-day domestic tasks such as cooking and personal hygiene and for family members to have adequate facilities and opportunity for sleep, for children to do school homework and for individuals to be able to have some privacy and time to themselves. Households that are subject to overcrowding, due to poor or inadequate housing, find it an up-hill battle to function effectively and to maintain healthy routines. Nor can they maintain their health and wellbeing without adequate food and appropriate nutrition. Even if people are capable of managing a sound diet and food preparation, they find it extraordinarily difficult in situations of overcrowding.

Access to affordable and nutritious food for families – especially in outback communities, is a problem that persists in many areas. There is evidence to suggest quite negative effects on mental health and child development due to inadequate or inappropriate nutrition; not to mention how this increases the risk of developing a range of chronic health conditions.

If we are genuine about suicide prevention, issues of housing and nutrition will need to be addressed with creative resolve. Examples of innovation in these areas do exist, but are not always generalisable. Solutions need to be developed and applied to individual communities.

If we are genuine about suicide prevention, issues of housing and nutrition will need to be addressed with creative resolve. Examples of innovation in these areas do exist, but are not always generalisable. Solutions need to be developed and applied to individual communities.

Supportive services for families rather than authoritarian interventions

Families in difficult circumstances need much support. Family wellbeing programs should not be generic, but tailored to the predominant issues and themes of families in individual Indigenous communities.

Appropriate services need to be provided to families that are most vulnerable and at risk, such as those with family members suffering from mental ill-health, particularly those with a prior history of self-harm, or a previous suicide attempt; where a family member has just been discharged from custody, or has a history of alcohol and drug abuse or domestic violence. Families in which there is a history of child neglect and abuse will need special monitoring and engagement and high level support.

Though the needs of these families may be obvious and even if services exist to support them, how these services are delivered and to what end, is of crucial importance.

So much more can be accomplished if service providers take a constructive genuinely concerned approach, rather than a routine or authoritarian one. The aims of such engagement should never result in perpetual clients or dependence, but recovery, self-management, resilience, social and emotional wellbeing. Even statutory agencies concerned with child abuse and neglect can take this approach, working on the basis not only of risk management and monitoring, but active family rehabilitation. Though these approaches may be enshrined in agency rhetoric, they don't always reflect in the attitudes and approach of agency workers.

So much more can be accomplished if service providers take a constructive genuinely concerned approach, rather than a routine or authoritarian one.

Even these approaches will fall short of what can be accomplished in families, without human service and statutory agencies themselves operating from a fully informed, integrated and interdisciplinary model of case management and care.

As already mentioned, ideally Indigenous community liaison workers, social and emotional wellbeing workers (common in Indigenous health services), can play a crucial role by working in close collaboration with counsellors, psychologists, mental health practitioners, community nurses, GPs, child protection and correctional and court services, in providing a seamless and comprehensive support for Indigenous families and family members. This does not require endless time wasting meetings, but merely some clear terms of reference, professional and effective communication, information sharing and constructive collaboration, out of respect and concern for what is in the best interests of clients.

Alcohol and substances

Family liaison and engagement, rather than conventional agency based responses, are needed for supporting families and family members experiencing the negative effects of alcohol and substance misuse.

Much more could be accomplished with local capacity of drug and alcohol counselling closely collaborating with other family support providers, such as social and emotional wellbeing and community liaison workers, health service staff, police and youth services. People that know and can work in and on behalf of their communities are most needed to stem the tide of problems flowing from alcohol and substance misuse.

The importance of these staff and other key concerned community individuals leading by example, especially when it comes to the responsible use of alcohol, should not be underestimated. Particularly young people are influenced much more by example than by merely being told to act responsibly. Much can be said for dealing with the issue of boredom of youth – especially in rural and remote communities, as a way of beginning to address the serious issues of alcohol and substance misuse in communities and all the problems – especially suicide, that these are associated with.

Particularly young people are influenced much more by example than by merely being told to act responsibly.

Conflict resolution and mediation skills training and support

Families that live in communities with poverty, social problems, high levels of distress, powerlessness and grief, are a breeding ground for conflict and violence, both within and between families. There is no substitute for properly addressing these social and community conditions, in order to diminish suicide risk and improve the overall health and wellbeing of families. However, there is still much to be gained by building capacity in families and communities by cultivating and training leaders and key community members in conflict management and mediation skills relevant to their cultural settings. There is much value and importance in building the skills and capacity of people who can work inside communities, with an intimate knowledge of individual families and the ability to read and manage the cultural nuances and cultural challenges involved.

Grief support and after suicide care of families and individuals

Access to grief and after suicide support for Indigenous families is often unavailable in many communities. Where grief and after suicide support is available from mainstream/non-Indigenous services, such support may not be adequately attuned to Indigenous understandings of and responses to bereavement, grief and mourning. The complexity here lies not only in understanding traditional local cultural beliefs and practices, but as well the different degrees to which Indigenous people subscribe to traditional beliefs and practices. For example, some people may participate in community rituals and responses, but may wish to be personally supported in a way that reflects a non-traditional or mainstream/non-Indigenous model of grief and mourning – including wanting to talk about the deceased person and engaging in a form of counselling that emphasises the importance of a developing biography of the deceased.

The complexity here lies not only in understanding traditional local cultural beliefs and practices, but as well the different degrees to which Indigenous people subscribe to traditional beliefs and practices.

Developing local competent capacity for responding to the enduring grief experienced by Indigenous communities as a result of suicide, needs to be addressed as a matter of priority.

Individual risk factors that may heighten the likelihood of suicide

- Experiencing alienation and anger
- High levels of psychological distress
- Psychological trauma from childhood or adult experiences
- Bereavement and grief overload
- Unemployment, underemployment, or lack of meaningful employment
- Death of a parent or child
- Lack of meaning and purpose
- Loss of cultural connections and identity
- Separation from a child, parent or sibling
- Experience of racism
- Exposure to self-harm and suicide behaviour
- Mental health difficulty that is not being adequately addressed
- Relationship separation: separated males, especially younger males, men who have experienced the breakdown of a marriage or de facto relationship and elderly widowed or divorced males, are particularly at risk of suicide
- Prior suicide attempt or prior history of repeated self-harm
- Recent discharge from custody or incarceration
- Drug or alcohol misuse
- Welfare dependence
- Family, intimate partner, sibling or elder violence
- Fear of reprisals and violence in inter-family disputes and conflict
- Fear of community violence – especially fear for the safety of children
- History or current experience of neglect or abuse

- Experience of and matters arising out of family law: such as child removal, custody dispute, relationship conflict, child access and support arrangements
- Poor health (such as chronic health condition)
- Conflicting sense of being 'caught between two cultures'
- Poverty – including lack of access to information, essential services, good nutrition and opportunities for improvement
- Over-exposure to and familiarity with death
- Poor housing and overcrowding
- Lack of family support or meaningful support network
- Issues of sexual identity and orientation: evidence suggests a correlation between gay men and suicide
- Experience of sexual assault or abuse
- Social disconnection and isolation – especially for men increases suicide risk
- Living in a rural or remote location
- Recent discharge from hospital having been admitted with a mental health difficulty
- Incarceration or recent release from incarceration
- Ready access to lethal means of suicide

Responding to Individual risk factors:

Improving service engagement with males

The majority of males at greatest risk of suicide are not successfully engaged by mental health services. Most male suicide victims who see their medical doctor prior to death (even on the day of their death) present solely with physical complaints. Plainly, the means by which suicidal thinking and pre-suicide distress are detected in patients is inadequate. Much of the problem is that health professionals often lack an understanding of the biology, psychology and cultural expectations that determine male experience and behaviour. Conflating suicidal experience and behaviour with mental 'illness' is problematic in a number of ways, not the least of which is that suicide is most often associated with psychological distress. To label this as an 'illness' is both unwarranted and potentially harmful to the person being labelled.

Much of the problem is that health professionals often lack an understanding of the biology, psychology and cultural expectations that determine male experience and behaviour.

Understanding powerlessness as a key issue for males

The significance of powerlessness particularly for males needs to be noted. The experience of powerlessness for males can give rise to a range of pronounced symptoms and behaviours, such as anger, psychological distress, mood disturbance, sleep disturbance or deprivation, anxiety, despondency, hopelessness, suicidal thoughts, aggression and risk taking, uncommunicativeness and social withdrawal.

Commonly, males who present in this way in primary care and mental health settings are unnecessarily and incorrectly diagnosed with depression, evidenced by the fact that when powerlessness or distress is identified and is even in a small way ameliorated, depressive symptoms and even suicidal thinking often quickly resolve.

Depression is sometimes associated with instances of male suicide. However, this should not be uncritically assumed, particularly with a male presentation of the kind described, without a proper and detailed assessment, and especially without first exploring the issue of powerlessness.

The experience and significance of powerlessness for males needs to be understood in relation to: male biology (specific physiology and endocrine mechanisms), the 'hardwired' action orientation of males (and their inherent need to be a cause that brings about an effect; a distinct need of a sense of personal agency and causality), socially and culturally reinforced male role expectations and the male need, particularly in the early adulthood, to achieve and maintain a favourable place in the male dominance hierarchy (a hierarchy amongst males which determines how individual males are viewed and valued by potential female reproductive partners).

Space does not permit a fuller explanation of these factors; suffice to say, they are real, potent and render men acutely vulnerable to the effects of experiencing powerlessness. When one considers the predicament of many Indigenous males today and their history of being subjugated, disenfranchised, demeaned, 'unmanned' and more recently, rendered dependent on welfare, it should not surprise us that being driven to extremes of distress, powerlessness and despair are commonly the circumstances of suicide.

When one considers the predicament of many Indigenous males today and their history of being subjugated, disenfranchised, demeaned, 'unmanned' and more recently, rendered dependent on welfare, it should not surprise us that being driven to extremes of distress, powerlessness and despair are commonly the circumstances of suicide.

Improved mental state and suicide risk assessment

Too often, individuals are shuffled in and out of busy service environments without adequate assessment. It is important that the mental health and suicide risk status of individuals are properly assessed in settings such as hospital accident and emergency departments where presentations for mental illness, trauma and substance abuse are common. Police responses to situations involving alcohol abuse, antisocial behaviour and violence requiring arrest and detention may need to be followed by assessment of risk of self-harm. Likewise, individuals being released from incarceration will need to be supported and engaged within a risk management framework. It is critically important that services and interventions are well-coordinated, information sharing and collaborative, culturally attuned and ensure clients have access to or are followed up by competent community-based preventive services.

Being watchful of older children and adolescents

In the general population, one in five young people (by current research estimates) will suffer from emotional problems and psychological distress sufficient to require professional support; this may be a conservative figure applied to Indigenous young people.

Adolescence especially is a time of great upheaval and change physically, physiologically, psychologically and socially. It can be a difficult and challenging time for young people, who may exhibit moodiness, changeability, impulsiveness, boundary testing and sensation seeking behaviours. They may go through times of being withdrawn, anxious and acting with too little concern for safety. They may also sometimes be difficult to live with, unreasonable and objectionable.

Though this may constitute a relatively normal profile of adolescent experience and behaviour, there are more pronounced 'stand out' signs of them beginning not to cope or running into serious trouble emotionally and psychologically, which might, if not addressed, put life itself at risk.

No-one can be expected to be a mind reader when it comes to discerning how a child or adolescent is coping. However, it is often possible to observe them more closely whenever there is the sense that perhaps they are doing more poorly than usual, are not coping in particular ways that are obvious and where there appears to be a cluster of ways in which they seem not to be coping. When there is concern, it is always best to ask them how they are coping (or to get someone else whom they trust to ask) and of course, if they are behaving in a way that is unsafe, or disclose that they are experiencing suicidal thoughts, immediate professional help should be sought. If such help isn't immediately available, then friends and family may need to close in around them, remain vigilant and try to keep them safe until professional help can be obtained. In the case of a young person expressing suicidal thoughts, or having engaged in significant self-harm, any lethal means of suicide will need to be removed from their environment.

One of the particular problems of youth suicide, which leaves surviving family and friends feeling so powerless and desolate, is that though some young people forecast their intentions to others, inviting the help and support they need, many others do not. They act impulsively, often under the influence of alcohol or drugs and leave their loved ones no opportunity to intervene.

One of the particular problems of youth suicide, which leaves surviving family and friends feeling so powerless and desolate, is that though some young people forecast their intentions to others, inviting the help and support they need, many others do not. They act impulsively, often under the influence of alcohol or drugs and leave their loved ones no opportunity to intervene.

There is no single factor that can be identified as most responsible for prompting young people to commit suicide, but research suggests that the more risk factors that are present, the more at-risk that person becomes. Of course, in individual cases some young people with multiple risk factors do not commit suicide and yet others with minimal risk factors will do so.

There is no sure means of prevention when it comes to child, adolescent or adult suicide. The best we can do is to endeavour to ensure that those we care about experience being valued, loved, heard, understood, known and emotionally and socially connected – which means keeping tabs not just on their behaviour but also on their emotional life. If they appear to be significantly distressed, or behave in ways that seem out of character or concerning, as best we can we need to let them know that someone cares and we need to try and connect them with a level of support and expertise that may help keep them safe and help them work through their problems.

Warning signs that young people might be in distress

- Becoming increasingly irritable, angry or hostile
- Getting into fights a lot
- Being often critical of, attacking and sarcastic to people around them
- Being frequently sad, tearful, with emotions appearing often to be 'close to the surface'
- Often listening to music that reflects hopelessness, anger, or despair
- Dressing in ways that reflect their sad or gloomy outlook and mood
- Decreased interest in getting out and doing things and appearing to derive little pleasure from previously enjoyable activities
- Withdrawing socially from friends and family; spending a lot of time alone, perhaps shut away and not communicating how they feel to anyone

- Disruptive behaviour at school and declining grades
- Frequent complaints of physical symptoms including: headaches, stomach aches, nausea, vomiting, dizziness and for girls, problems with menstruation
- Expressing boredom and disinterest and exhibiting a lack of motivation much of the time
- An intense preoccupation with their weight or body image
- Excessive or compulsive exercising
- Concerning degree of risk-taking and sensation-seeking
- Showing little interest in personal hygiene or appearance
- Expressing that they are a failure, can't do anything and have a negative view of their own self-worth and their value to others
- Blaming themselves for negative events or circumstances, or being blamed for a death or something bad that has happened to someone else; which may emanate from cultural/spiritual beliefs used to provide an explanation for what has happened
- Frequently appearing highly stressed, anxious, uptight, tense, agitated or panicky
- Being deeply pessimistic and negative about the future
- A major change in sleeping patterns: being tired during the day, not being able to get to sleep or not being able to stay asleep sufficient to wake refreshed
- A major change in eating patterns: a developing pattern of comfort eating resulting in weight gain, or a loss of appetite resulting in loss of weight
- Abuse of alcohol or one or more of a range of substances available in the community
- Preoccupation with someone they know that has committed suicide
- Talk of running away from home or actually running away even for a short time
- A decline in their usual preparedness to communicate and a tendency to become secretive
- Intense preoccupation with a broken relationship
- A tendency to go over and over their experience and thoughts in their mind; or experiencing intrusive thoughts which interrupt their concentration at school or at home
- An inability to calm powerful emotions, so that their experience is often dominated by these emotions, which impedes their ability to think rationally about things

- Showing tell-tale signs of self-harm or disclosing to someone that they self-harm
- Talk of life not being worthwhile, of not wanting to be around anymore, or of ending their life

Male and female similarities and differences

Very little research has sought to clarify the gender specific ways in which men and women display the kind of inability to cope and other signs of distress or psychological difficulty that might lead to suicide. In general we can say that men and women may exhibit distress and emotional and psychological difficulties in a number of similar ways. However, they (especially men) sometimes display no clear signs or symptoms of difficulty and may not reach out to anyone for help or support.

Women are much more accustomed to help-seeking than men, they can more readily find support services suited to their needs and their help-seeking is culturally encouraged rather than disparaged as it is for men. Especially under stress, women are more likely to communicate their experience and seek social connection for support. Men tend to adopt a different coping style to women and are not usually so emotionally or verbally expressive of their experience. However, they do often reach out (in a way suited to their coping style) to male friends or peers – especially in circumstances that afford a reassuring sense of emotional safety, or in environments that are all-male. Unfortunately, such opportunities are not always readily available for men and they can be left to deal with their distress in isolation – which may put them at greater risk.

Women are much more accustomed to help-seeking than men, they can more readily find support services suited to their needs and their help-seeking is culturally encouraged rather than disparaged as it is for men.

It should not be assumed, based on male suicide statistics, that males cope more poorly than females; this isn't supported by mental health incidence or prevalence data, or by what we know about on-average gender specific styles of coping. What we do know is that males tend to approach suicide with greater decisiveness and often using more lethal means; another reason why we need to be much more proactive in relation to male suicide prevention.

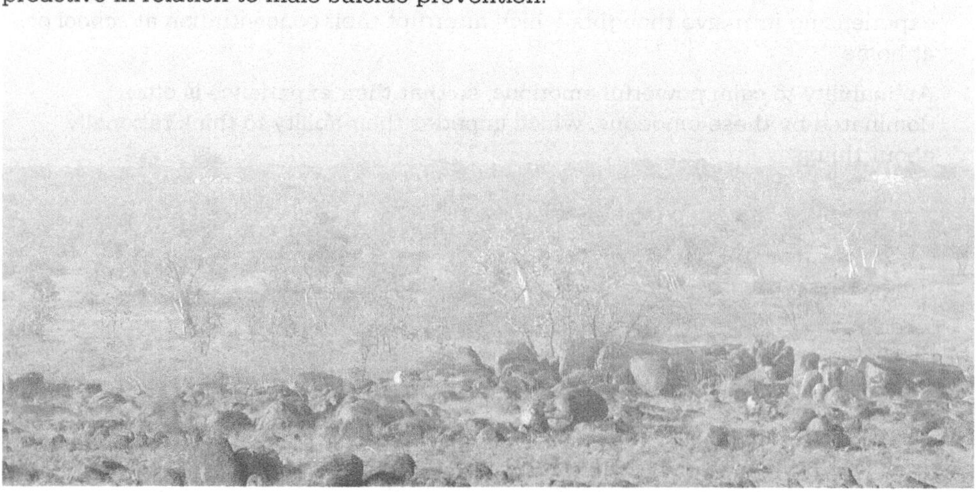

Warning signs that adults might be in distress

- Displaying distress, anxiety and appearing to be overwhelmed by things
- Becoming uncommunicative, secretive, distant and/or preoccupied
- Not coping with work or day to day living
- Showing signs of being exhausted, fatigued and/or despondent
- Not mixing socially as usual; neglecting family and friends; appearing to withdraw into his/her own world and experience
- Difficulties with sleep: getting to sleep, staying asleep, or not getting enough sleep
- Changed eating habits: either not hungry or overeating
- Irritable, gets easily upset, angry, argumentative and/or blows up over little things
- Talks about being really stressed and looks visibly stressed and 'wound up'
- Drinking more heavily, or has begun using substances more frequently
- Personal appearance and self-care are deteriorating
- Appears to lack motivation; loss of interest in things usually found enjoyable
- Appears quite intense and panicky and seems to be driven and attempting to do far too much at one time
- Struggling to make choices and appears paralysed in decision making
- Engaging in risky and careless behaviour (such as drink driving or speeding)
- Letting things pile up and leaving things undone
- Appears to be ignoring an important relationship issue
- Seems to be acting strangely, or out of character
- Is in financial difficulties, but is either ignoring the problem, or is overwhelmed with worry
- Talks about being useless and says "my family would be better off without me"
- Seems to be coldly and efficiently putting everything in order, but is not communicating with others and seems numb and without feeling
- Has mentioned that life is not worth the effort and that everything always goes wrong
- Being often critical of, attacking and sarcastic to other people
- Being frequently sad, tearful, with emotions appearing often to be 'close to the surface'

- Decreased interest in getting out and doing things
- Withdrawing socially from friends and family; spending a lot of time alone, perhaps shut away and not communicating
- Frequent complaints of physical symptoms including: headaches, stomach aches, nausea, back pain, muscular pain and light-headedness
- Expressing that they are a failure, can't do anything and have a negative view of their own self-worth and their value to others
- Blaming themselves for negative events or circumstances, or being blamed for a death or something bad that has happened to someone else; which may emanate from cultural/spiritual beliefs used to provide an explanation for what has happened
- Frequently appearing highly stressed, anxious, uptight, tense and agitated
- Being deeply pessimistic and negative about the future
- Intense preoccupation with a broken relationship
- A tendency to go over and over their experience and thoughts in their mind; or experiencing intrusive thoughts which interrupt their concentration
- An inability to calm powerful emotions, so that their experience is often dominated by these emotions, which impedes their ability to think rationally about things
- Talk of life not being worthwhile, of not wanting to be around anymore, or of ending their life

Helping someone who is experiencing suicidal thoughts – *things to bear in mind*

- Negotiate to take charge of any readily available means for acting on suicidal thoughts or impulses, such as guns, knives, rope, pills, or car keys (if you think a vehicle might be used). You may need to be insistent about this, particularly if your sense is that the person is at high risk.
- Remember *you are not responsible* for someone else's suicidal behaviour. You have no control over their will. If they choose to act in a self-harming or destructive way, *they* have chosen to do so; *they* are ultimately responsible, not anyone who is trying to help and support them.
- Talking to a person about suicidal thoughts *won't* encourage them to act on them, but will signal genuine concern and an avenue of hope.
- Think about how best to approach the person, given what you know about their personality and temperament; be determined but respectful.

- A person experiencing suicidal thoughts may not be easy to help. They may be so distressed or troubled that they see everything as pointless, except putting an end to how they are feeling. You may need to persevere. The most important thing will be to ensure their safety.
- If you don't think they'll listen to you, then consider who else they usually confide in, feel comfortable with and/or trust. Maybe this person could make the approach and encourage them to seek assistance. Provide them with the 24/7 Crisis Line number (see the list towards the end of this resource). Follow up to see if things worked out.
- You yourself can seek advice and guidance about what to do at any time, by calling a mental health crisis line number in your State (see the list).

Practical tips on how to help

- Try to create opportunities – safe and private occasions where you can ask about the person about their experience – how they are really experiencing things. If you don't ask, you won't know. However, don't delay waiting for the 'perfect occasion'; their safety is all important.
- Listen to them and their experience attentively, with an open mind and without judgement. With a man, don't expect him to use the kind of feeling words that women use. Women may be verbally and emotionally expressive, but men tend to use action metaphors to communicate their emotion experience: "I've fallen in a hole lately"; "things have been getting me down"; "I'm struggling to stay afloat"; I've been dragging my feet".
- If the person has strong distressing feelings, acknowledge and validate them: "sounds like things are really hard for you at present?", or, "feeling like you do can't be easy, how about we put our heads together and see what can be done to help?"
- Affirm the person's value and worth and that they are needed and wanted.
- Find ways to help them engage more socially and to better connect with positive family and friends.
- Drop in on them unexpectedly; this can sometimes help to break their pattern of self-defeating thoughts.
- With a man, consider offering to work alongside him in some way, like doing something in his yard; maybe invite him to become involved with you in a recreational activity, like fishing, hunting, or going bush for a while, or some other physical activity (physical activity and 'putting his head in a better place', can be very helpful).
- With a woman, consider a good way of involving her socially and spend time with her to provide an opportunity for her to talk about how she is feeling, what is happening in her life

- Explain how alcohol is a depressant and makes things much worse, rather than being of any genuine relief. The person you are trying to help may also benefit from knowing that, though alcohol appears to help sleep – because it helps people fall asleep more easily, it actually degrades the quality of sleep – again making coping all the harder. Explain that alcohol can significantly fuel suicidal thinking.
- If the person has become withdrawn and inactive, encourage them to become active again. Helping them set some small achievable daily goals may help them start to feel in control of life again.
- If the person is very anxious and restless, encourage them to cut caffeine out of their diet by finding de-caffeinated substitutes. Caffeine makes anxiety much worse and it degrades sleep.
- With a man, encourage him to try and explain the way(s) in which he might feel powerless or overwhelmed. Sometimes, doing even some small thing that can help alleviate a man's sense of powerlessness can make a big difference to his experience. A small *act of power* or problem solving initiative can be a powerful antidote to powerlessness.
- Get the person to think about what is worthwhile and precious in their life and who depends upon and values them.
- Talk to the person about the terrible impact that suicide has on others – and that sometimes they never recover from its effects.
- Try to get the person to promise not to harm themselves and to accept assistance.
- You will need to convey that you're seriously concerned. Suggest to the person that they talk confidentially to a counsellor or mental health practitioner, immediately. Follow up to see how this turned out. Or, if you think they might be unsafe, suggest that they see a doctor immediately, go to a hospital, or local outback clinic, or that they ring the 24/7 Mental Health Crisis Line (see the list towards the end of this resource). Offer to help them to make the phone call or to attend the appointment. Always follow up to see how things turned out.
- Get agreement for you to remove all means that are immediately available to the person for committing suicide. This includes guns (the police can remove these and keep them until a person has recovered and is safe) pills, poison, rope and car and truck keys (if you think vehicles might be used).
- Try and conscript the help of relatives or friends to keep a watchful eye on the person, to break their isolation and to provide extra safety.
- If the person appears determined to act on their suicidal thoughts and especially if they have the means and a plan and they won't seek and accept immediate assistance, call the police. **Better to lose a friend than for a person to lose their life.**

A person experiencing suicidal thoughts needs to hear a number of important things

- No matter how bad your situation, no matter how overwhelming your mental/emotional pain, there is always a better option than considering suicide – but it may not have occurred to you. Speak to a doctor, go to a hospital or local clinic, or phone the 24/7 Mental Health Crisis Line; help and relief can quickly follow.
- A person who kills themselves does terrible violence to their family and friends. Thinking "they'd be better off without me" doesn't cancel out the fact that they'd be greatly damaged – perhaps for life. Promise yourself (and someone else) that you'll get help; that you'll do it now and you won't give up until you get it.
- Suicidal thinking is often driven by a state of ongoing deep or acute distress. This shouldn't be ignored. A person doesn't have to be depressed to be suicidal. Anxiety is also independently associated with suicide. Seek help immediately.
- Who are the people that really matter to you? Think about why they matter and the good things that have happened between you.
- If you have a gun, rope, pills, or anything else you've thought of using to kill yourself, either lock them up and give the key to someone for safe keeping, or hand them over to someone, so that you're kept from harm's way until you've received help and have recovered.
- Feelings of hopelessness, helplessness and overwhelming mental/emotional pain can be quickly turned around with appropriate assistance and support
- Things can be made to feel and look very different; hope for the future can be restored, if you act with courage and speak to a doctor, go to a hospital, or phone the 24/7 Mental Health Crisis Line.

'We may not have control over many things that happen to us, but we can always choose how we will respond'

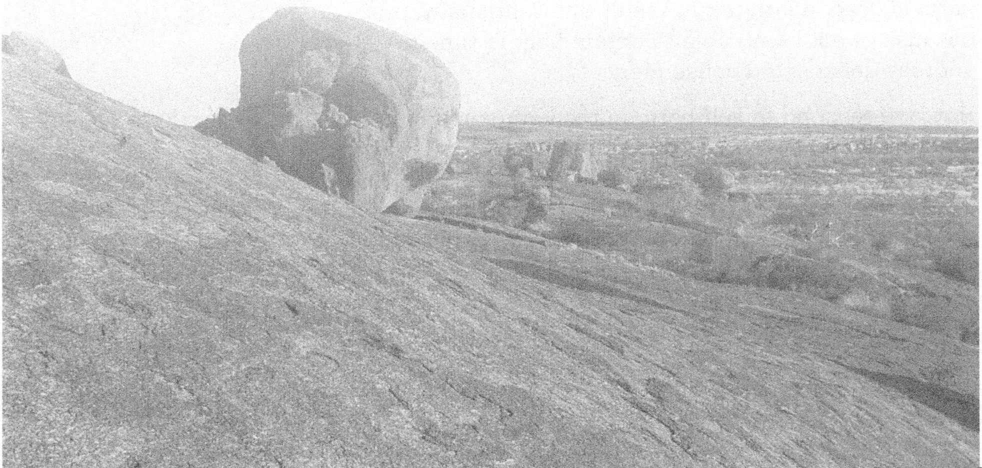

Teenagers and self-harm in Indigenous communities

Self-harm is becoming increasingly common

Teenage self-harm is now a common problem seen by many teachers, school counsellors, mental health workers, psychologists and psychotherapists. It is a problem that has significantly increased over the last several decades and is most common amongst females. From the outset it is important to realise that it is much more complex and potentially serious than mere juvenile attention seeking.

Though it is often triggered by experiences like bullying, or difficulties in relationships at home or with peers, it appears most fundamentally associated with struggling to regulate strong emotions – being unable to change or manage an overwhelming or unpleasant emotion state.

Another reason not to be hasty in thinking that self-harm is just another behaviour of immature youth, is that adults too are known to engage in this behaviour, many of whom likewise struggle with emotion management. Furthermore, adults use all kinds of equally unhelpful means of escaping or ameliorating unwanted emotion states, such as alcohol, prescribed and illicit substances, food, cigarettes, gambling and even 'retail therapy', yet none of these tend to attract the same stigma and are mostly culturally acceptable.

Self-harm should be taken seriously

Though many teenagers who self-harm may not have a desire to kill themselves, such behaviour may still express a powerful state of despair – which needs to be taken seriously. And, though self-harm is most often not suicidal behaviour, with practice it makes suicide potentially a less foreign and statistically more likely behaviour.

Some research suggests that self-harm can be a stronger predictor of a future suicide attempt than a prior suicide attempt in adolescents with depression.

Another factor is that if a dangerous method of self-harm is used, death might result unintentionally, or because of not being able to obtain help in time to address unexpected consequences.

How we respond to self-harm in teenagers needs to be thoughtful, decisive and appropriate to their particular circumstances, experience and background issues. Our response must be one that ensures safety at the same time as avoiding overreaction – which can cause shame and embarrassment and may discourage future help-seeking.

Our response must be one that ensures safety at the same time as avoiding overreaction – which can cause shame and embarrassment and may discourage future help-seeking.

What is self-harm?

Self-harm is any behaviour where the intent is to deliberately cause harm to oneself. It may involve scratches through to deep wounds requiring sutures, or burns requiring medical treatment. Self-harm can be a transient behaviour that is triggered by particular stressful events – and which resolves relatively quickly, or a longer term theme of behaviour that is associated with a more serious psychological or mental health disorder. It may begin as a mild repetitive behaviour which increasingly becomes a habitual way of responding to emotional discomfort or distress.

Methods of self-harm may include:

- Cutting or burning oneself
- Skin picking, hair pulling, or head banging
- Taking an overdose of tablets
- Swallowing hazardous materials or substances
- Over/under-medicating (such as insulin)
- Punching or hitting oneself
- Abusing alcohol or some other substance
- Over/under-eating
- Driving recklessly
- Having unsafe sex

Why do teenagers self-harm?

There are many factors that motivate teenagers to self-harm, including the need to express and escape from deep emotional distress and pain, or a situation they experience as unbearable. Self-harm can be a way of coping with feelings of sadness, self-loathing, emptiness, guilt or rage. It may in some cases be a way of inducing caring and concern in others.

Self-harm can create permission to withdraw from social responsibility and the heavily felt expectations of others by creating a 'sick role', or by attracting a mental illness diagnosis, which unfortunately is often too hastily applied to teenagers on being sent to the family doctor or some other health professional.

Self-harm can be an act of power – a way of experiencing personal agency *(I exist, I matter and I can make things happen)*, which may be absent from other areas of a teenager's life – especially if their experience of adults is mostly demanding and commanding. It can be a way of expressing feeling that can't be put into words, or of feeling *something* rather than just feeling numb.

However, one can never and should never assume the motive for self-harm, because it may also be because a person does actually want to kill themselves.

However, one can never and should never assume the motive for self-harm, because it may also be because a person does actually want to kill themselves.

As counterintuitive as it may seem, self-harm can help a person feel better, despite possibly being quite painful. If it didn't help in some way it wouldn't be used. Not only can *wounding pain,* like cutting or burning, shift an emotion state, it also prompts the release of endorphins which have a soothing effect; endorphins are a natural pain reliever that gives temporary relief and a sense of peace. The addictive nature of this feeling can make stopping self-harm difficult.

The down side of self-harm

One of the major drawbacks of self-harm as a modifier of emotion experience is that it doesn't deal with the issues that prompted its use in the first place. When used as a method of managing emotion experience, in the absence of more helpful ways of learning to respond to the inevitable difficulties of daily life, it can become a stubborn compulsion that is difficult to budge.

Short term relief of self-harm is often followed by feeling ashamed and guilty, which encourages secretiveness and isolation. Keeping self-harm a secret from family and friends can be both difficult and lonely. It can also be dangerous, where the effects of some forms of self-harm are underestimated.

Keeping self-harm a secret from family and friends can be both difficult and lonely. It can also be dangerous, where the effects of some forms of self-harm are underestimated.

Inevitably, secretiveness tends to foster suspicion in friends and family, with the potential to negatively affect relationships. The alarm and reaction of parents to discovering that their teenager is self-harming and their tendency not to differentiate it from attempted or rehearsed suicide, can result in a strong reaction and a sometimes escalating drama of interventions that leave the teenager feeling publicly exposed, highly embarrassed and socially alienated from their peers, who may quickly label them as mentally disturbed or strange.

This can all lead to feeling even more lonely, worthless and trapped.

Myths about self-harm

Lots of misconceptions exist about self-harm (whether it involves cutting or some other means) – especially about a teenager's motives and mental state.

Myth: Self-harm is just to get attention

The fact is, in most cases self-harm is done in secret and to parts of the body (such as with cutting and burning) that are hidden from view – such as thighs, upper arms or abdomen. Should self-harm be used for inducing caring and concern in others, or even if it appears quite minor in method and something occurring amongst peers in a group, professional advice should still be sought without delay.

Myth: Teenagers who self-harm are mentally ill

Whilst some teenagers who self-harm do suffer from some degree of anxiety or depression, or as a result of psychological trauma, this should never be assumed. And anyway, some degree of anxiety and depression is common in the general population and in individual cases is only considered a problem if it is sufficiently severe. Many teenagers who self-harm have no discernible major mental health difficulty. More often than not they are struggling with difficult developmental or life issues and emotion regulation and need competent assistance to develop the skill and capacity to tackle and manage these.

Myth: If the self-harm is only minor it shouldn't be considered serious

Whether self-harm is serious or not for any individual teenager is something that should never be assumed and should be thoughtfully and carefully assessed by someone competent to do so. One must still carefully consider the underlying goal of the self-harming behaviour and what is happing in the life and experience of the teenager using this behaviour. Though self-harm may begin in a minor way, it can become habitual, addictive and more dangerous as time goes on.

Myth: If they've secretly been self-harming they won't want to disclose it

This may be the case, but should never be assumed. If someone shows them care with calm, is not judgmental and does not intend to betray their trust, they may in fact be relieved to be able to tell someone about not only their self-harm but what they are experiencing that has prompted it. Caring acceptance without judgement is more often than not a great door opener and can lead to a person not only feeling valued and understood, but also being amenable to accepting help.

Myth: Teenagers that self-harm are from dysfunctional lower socioeconomic families

The use of self-harm to manage emotional distress is common in affluent *and* poorer neighbourhoods and families. It is no respecter of social class or standing and it is common in both non-Indigenous and Indigenous families and communities.

Warning signs of self-harm

Clothing can of course hide physical injuries and emotional pain can be covered over with a deceptive public mask. Nevertheless, warning signs that a teenager is self-harming may become evident. There are signs you can look for and you don't have to be sure that a teenager is self-harming to reach out to them if you are worried. If they are unreceptive to your approach, you may be able to ask someone they confide in or trust to enquire about how they are. And sometimes it can be helpful to be specific in asking about how things are going at home, at school, with their peers, their study, or in dealing with an issue you know they are facing. Warning signs of self-harm might include:

There are signs you can look for and you don't have to be sure that a teenager is self-harming to reach out to them if you are worried.

- Unexplained cuts, bruises, burns, or abrasions
- A tendency to always want to keep their arms, thighs, or abdomen covered even in hot weather
- Secretiveness – spending long periods of time in the bathroom or bedroom
- Changes in eating and sleeping habit
- Blood stains on clothing, towels, bedding or tissues
- Explaining frequent 'accidents' by saying "I'm just clumsy"
- Carrying in their belongings means of self-harm, like razor blades, a shard of glass, needles, sharp metal, or a cigarette lighter, or some form of acid
- Withdrawal from friends and family
- Using alcohol or drugs
- Expressing a feeling of failure, uselessness, or a loss of hope
- Lowering of academic performance
- Becoming increasingly irritable and aggressive
- Talking of self-harm or suicide
- Giving away personal possessions

Risk factors

A number of factors can make a teenager vulnerable to self-harm and these often exist in combination. Factors may include:

- Inability to adequately express or put into words significant emotions and emotion experience
- Low self-confidence and poor self-image
- Experiencing a sense of powerlessness, being trapped and having little sense of control
- Alcohol and drug misuse

- Poor problem solving skills
- A tendency to be impulsive
- Anxiety and/or a persistent downturn in mood
- Loneliness or isolation
- Feeling different and being seen as different (in a negative way)
- Conflict at home with parents or siblings
- Violence in the family at home
- Family is in conflict with another family in the community
- Mental health difficulty, self-harm or suicide in the family
- Expression of emotion in the family is discouraged
- Neglect, or physical, sexual or emotional abuse
- Separated, divorced or warring parents
- Unreasonable family expectations
- Difficulty in relationships and in relating to others
- Easy access to drugs, medication, or other means of self-harm
- Experience of racism
- Bullying and/or peer rejection or social exclusion

Cycle of self-harm

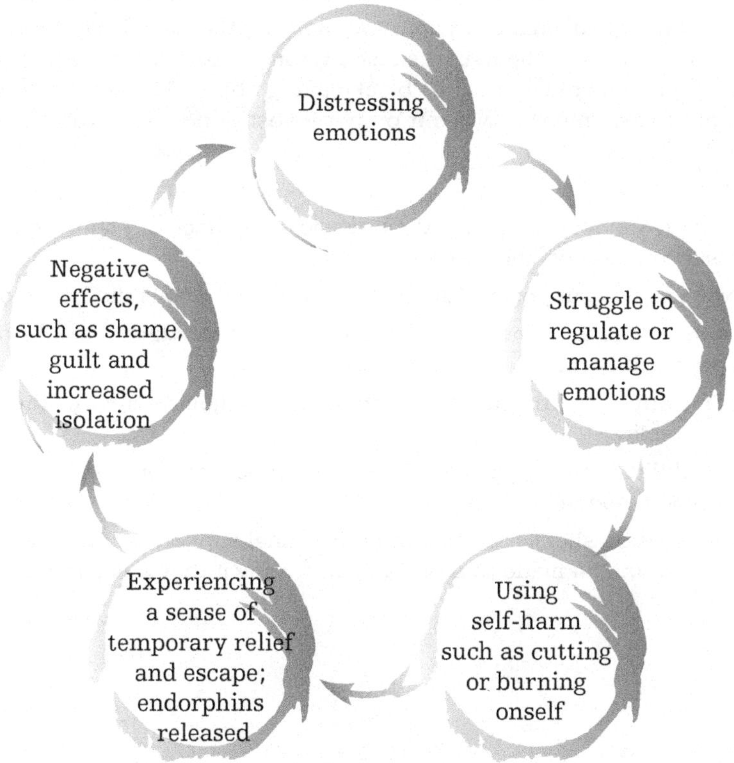

Self-harm versus suicidal behaviour

As already mentioned, though many teenagers who self-harm may not have a desire to kill themselves, such behaviour may still express a powerful state of despair – which needs to be taken seriously. Though self-harm is most often not suicidal behaviour, with practice it makes suicide potentially a less foreign and statistically more likely behaviour. And as some research suggests, in the case of adolescents with depression, it can be a stronger predictor of a future suicide attempt than a prior suicide attempt.

Despite this worrying correlation between self-harm and suicide, it is important not to confuse or conflate the two. There are several reasons for this:

- Though self-harm should be risk-managed to prevent escalation and increased danger, our response to suicidal thinking and suicidal behaviour tends to be much more assertive and less concerned about protecting the privacy or confidentiality of the individual.
- It is the commonly held view of health professionals that the personal autonomy of individuals who disclose suicidal thinking – and especially suicidal intention, should be considered secondary to a duty of care and responsibility to intervene protectively.
- Responding to self-harm with the same degree of intervention applied to suicide – unless the nature of the self-harm is life threatening or dangerous in nature and implication, may be an overreaction with potential to put a teenager using self-harm with no suicidal intent at greater risk; not only due to precipitating anger and resentment towards service providers, but also by thrusting the teenager into a place of diminished amenability to seeking assistance in future.
- When self-harm and suicidal behaviour are merged, there is also potential for teenagers to leverage the fear of suicide wrongly associated with minor self-harm, as a means of emotionally blackmailing adults. However it is very important not to assume this without proper investigation and professional advice.

If a teenager is in the process of self-harming, here are some ways of responding:

- Remain calm, avoid overreaction and expressions of shock or anger (remember self-harm is a common coping mechanism)
- Express concern and support for them, not judgement about the behaviour
- Avoid trivialising the issue or situation that the teenager thinks may have triggered their self-harm
- Ask if there is anything you can do to help alleviate their distress or the 'bad' way they are feeling
- Consider carefully if any medical attention is needed and discuss with them what you think is needed
- Begin a conversation about the value of professional support and reassure them that every effort will be made to protect their privacy if they will accept support

If you suspect a teenager has been injuring themselves, here are some ways of responding:

- Deal with your own feelings first: you may feel shocked, embarrassed, disappointed, or angry. By acknowledging your own experience, you will likely be more capable of remaining calm and showing concern and support
- Before you express concern, be sure to prepare yourself for the possibility of hearing things that you may not be comfortable hearing
- Create an opportunity of privacy and express your concern calmly and without judgment. People who self-harm often already feel shame and embarrassment.
- Offer support, not any kind of ultimatum or punishment
- Encourage them to talk about whatever it is that they think might be fuelling or triggering their self-harming behaviour
- Put the focus of attention on their understanding of their experience and the circumstances that have led to self-harm, rather than their injuries
- Begin a conversation about the value of professional support and reassure them that every effort will be made to protect their privacy if they will accept support

When decisiveness is required

- In the case of a teenager disclosing suicidal thoughts, professional intervention should be sought immediately.
- If a teenager has harmed themselves by taking an overdose of medication or consuming poison, call an ambulance to avoid any risk of permanent harm or the risk of death. It is of vital importance to identify as accurately as possible the name of the medication, poison or substance used, for assessment by the medical staff.
- First aid may be sought for minor injuries, where a qualified first aid person can also decide whether referral to a doctor is required.
- For any major injury, medical assistance should be sought, whether from a local medical clinic, GP, hospital accident and emergency, or a flying doctor or paramedical service. It is usually possible to gain immediate and sound advice by telephone in conversation with these service providers.
- In any circumstance where it is disclosed or evident that a teenager is at real risk of suicide, has perhaps attempted suicide, or has suicidal intent, professional intervention should be sought immediately.
- In any circumstance where a teenager discloses suicidal thinking and especially intent, or appears to have attempted suicide and yet is unwilling to seek or accept immediate assistance, it is best to initiate an intervention that does not require their consent. This can be done by calling the Police. In circumstances where no police are available (such as in a remote community) improvised action by concerned adults until police assistance arrives may be necessary.

Seeking professional help

Whether or not to seek professional help for a teenager engaging in self-harm is a delicate matter and is really about exercising careful consideration. Certainly, avoiding seeking help due to embarrassment, or not wanting to divulge 'family business' may, in a case of potential escalation of the behaviour, be putting the teenager at further risk. In the case of minor self-harm there may be less urgency in seeking professional intervention. However, it is usually advisable to at least begin a conversation with a health professional for a collaborative monitoring of the situation and to pick up on and respond to any signs of escalation in the behaviour. Early intervention is always better than having to deal later with a more entrenched pattern of self-harm.

Much care and thought needs to go into encouraging a teenager to accept help and to ensuring the very best arrangements for their privacy and ease of access to sessions. Arranging session times that clash with favourite classes at school, a valued recreational activity, or that jeopardise an important work commitment or routine, will only likely serve as a discouragement to attend sessions and to engage with them helpfully.

Psychotherapy for emotion regulation problems and self-harm

There is still a lack of research about the most effective psychotherapies for emotion regulation difficulties and self-harm and so there are gaps in our knowledge. Some of the psychotherapies that have been found to be helpful include: Acceptance and Commitment Therapy, Mindfulness, Dialectical Behavioural Therapy, Gestalt Therapy, Cognitive Behavioural Therapy and Existential Psychotherapy. This is by no means a comprehensive list of potential psychotherapies, nor should too much emphasis be placed on them anyway, since robust research in the field of *common factors contributing to positive outcomes in therapy* suggests that the type of psychotherapy used by a helping professional or program is far less significant than the therapeutic relationship the helping professional can foster with the client.

Because of how much courage it can take for a teenager to talk about their experience and confide in a therapist, it is vitally important to ensure that the psychotherapist or psychologist selected has a good track record of building rapport with teenagers, can offer consistent and reliable availability of sessions (if needed) and is willing to collaborate and consult with school staff, parents and the teenager's GP, should that be important to achieving the best outcome for the teenage client.

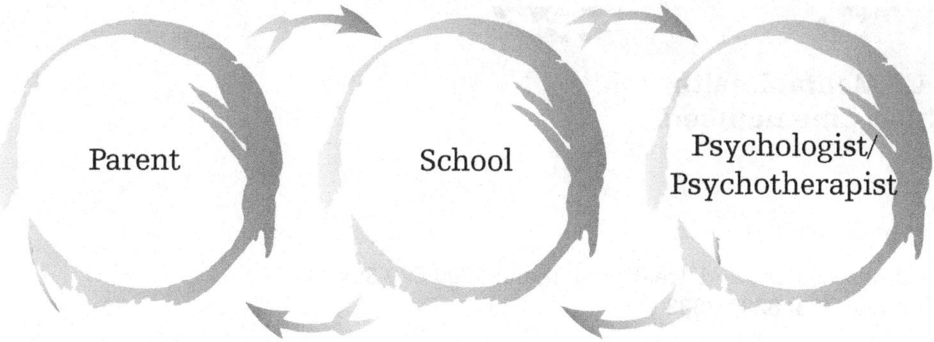

Working together

Ideally, significant adults concerned about a teenager who is self-harming will discuss and agree on the best approach to take and continue to communicate to ensure consistency and to review progress. Reasonable and circumstantial obstacles can get in the way of this but, suffice to say, it is important for helpers not to be acting at cross purposes, but to be part of an effective concerted effort.

Where to get help if someone is having thoughts of suicide

Emergency

For immediate assistance when life may be in danger
Call 000
Suicide Callback Service – emergency

Lifeline

13 11 14 – 24/7 hotline
Crisis Support and Suicide Prevention services
www.lifeline.org.au

Suicide Call Back Service

1300 659 467 – 24/7 hotline
The Suicide Call Back Service provides free nationwide professional telephone and online counselling for anyone affected by suicide.

Beyond Blue

1300 22 4636 – 24/7 hotline
Depression. Anxiety. Talk it through with us, day or night
www.beyondblue.org.au

Headspace

National Youth Mental Health Foundation providing early intervention mental health services to 12 – 25 year olds: 1800 063 267

Kids Help Line

1800 55 1800
For ages 5 – 25 years
www.kidshelp.com.au

Mens Line

1300 78 99 78
MensLine Australia is a professional telephone and online support and information service for Australian men.
www.mensline.org.au

24/7 Mental Health Crisis Line numbers

Australian Capital Territory

Crisis Assessment and Treatment Team: 1800 629 354
Parentline: (02) 6287 3833

New South Wales

NSW Mental Health Line 1800 011 511
Parentline: 1300 1300 52

Northern Territory

Mental Health Access Team: 1800 682 288
Parentline: 1300 30 1300

Queensland

Parentline: 1300 30 1300

South Australia

Mental Health Assessment and Crisis Intervention Service: 13 14 65
Parent Helpline: 1300 364 100

Tasmania

Mental Health Services Helpline: 1800 332 388; Parenting Line: 1300 808 178

Victoria

Mental Health Advice Line: 1300 280 737; SuicideLine: 1300 651 251;
Parentline: 13 22 89

Western Australia

Mental Health Emergency Response Line: Metro 1300 555 788;
Rural Link: Rural 1800 552 002; Parenting Line: 1800 654 43

Self-Harm – pathways to help and support

General Practitioner

General Medical Practitioners play a crucial role in their communities in monitoring and maintaining the health of families. This familiarity makes them often the trusted 'first port of call' for physical injury or issues of mental health.

Most GPs do not routinely prescribe medication such as antidepressants to teenagers, since it is always preferable to explore other approaches and psychotherapy before considering medication. They can provide referral to subsidised psychology and mental health services of the Primary Care Networks and may know trusted private psychotherapy or psychology practitioners whom they can recommend.

Before requesting a GP referral to other subsidised services, it is best to discuss whether this entails needing a mental health plan. Such a plan does require a diagnosis, which some people find undesirable due to perceived stigma.

Headspace: youth counselling and mental health services

Headspace is the National Youth Mental Health Foundation providing early intervention mental health services to 12-25 year olds.

No GP referral or mental health plan is required to access this service. Teenagers can self-refer and parents and teachers can seek free advice.

The service is designed to make it as easy as possible for a young person and their family to get the help they need for problems affecting their wellbeing. This covers four core areas: mental health, physical health, work and study support and alcohol and other drug services. Headspace centres are located across metropolitan, regional and rural areas of Australia. Centres are built and designed with input from young people so they don't have the same look or feel as other clinical services.

They are there so that young people can access the type of health worker they need.

This could be a GP, psychologist, social worker, alcohol and drug worker, counsellor, vocational worker or youth worker. A number of centres also have Aboriginal and Torres Strait Islander health workers, welfare workers and family therapists.

To find a headspace centre near you, go to:

www.headspace.org.au/headspace-centres, or phone: 03 9027 0100

Primary Health Networks and Psychology and Mental Health services

These networks fund psychology and mental health services in many locations across Australia – including outreach into regional and rural locations. Services are subsidised by the Federal Government and may be offered free or attracting a gap payment.

Though immediate access may in some locations be limited due to waiting lists, these services are often prepared to give priority to teenagers with issues of a serious nature. These services may require a GP referral and mental health plan. Such a plan will include a diagnosis, which some people may find undesirable due to perceived stigma.

To find Primary Health Network funded services near you, simply Google: PHN Map Locator and select your area. If you have any difficulty locating a Primary Health Network that covers your area, email phn@health.gov.au

References used in the preparation of this resource

Aldridge, D., et al. (2012) 'Psychotherapeutic approaches to non-suicidal self-injury in adolescents', *Child and Adolescent Psychiatry and Mental Health* 6:14.

Arsenault-Lapierre, G., Kim, C. & Turecki, G. (Nov 2004) 'Psychiatric diagnoses in 3275 suicides: a meta-analysis', *BMC Psychiatry* 4: 37.

Asarnow, J.R., et al. (2011) 'Suicide attempts and non-suicidal self-injury in the treatment of resistant depression in adolescents: findings from the TORDIA study', *Journal of the American Academy of Child and Adolescent Psychiatry* 50:8, 772-781.

Ashfield, J. (2011) *Doing Psychotherapy with Men: Practicing Ethical Psychotherapy and Counselling with Men*. Australian Institute of Male Health and Studies.

Ashfield, J., Smith, A. & Bain, L. (2015) *Preventing Male Suicide: Become Part of the Solution*. Australian Institute of Male Health and Studies. See www.aimhs.com.au

Ashfield, J. (2015) *Teenagers and Self-harm: What Every Parent and Teacher Needs to Know*. YouCanHelp Training for Life, Australia. See www.youcanhelp.com.au

Ashfield, J. (2004) *The Nature of Men: Elements of Masculine Psychology*. Australia: Mid North Regional Health Service.

Australian Bureau of Statistics. (2015). *Causes of Death, Australia, 2012*. Catalogue No. 3303.0. Belconnen, ACT: Commonwealth of Australia. Accessed March 31, 2015

Australian Bureau of Statistics. (2013). *Causes of Death, Australia, 2011*. Catalogue No. 3303.0. Belconnen, ACT: Commonwealth of Australia. Accessed March 25, 2014

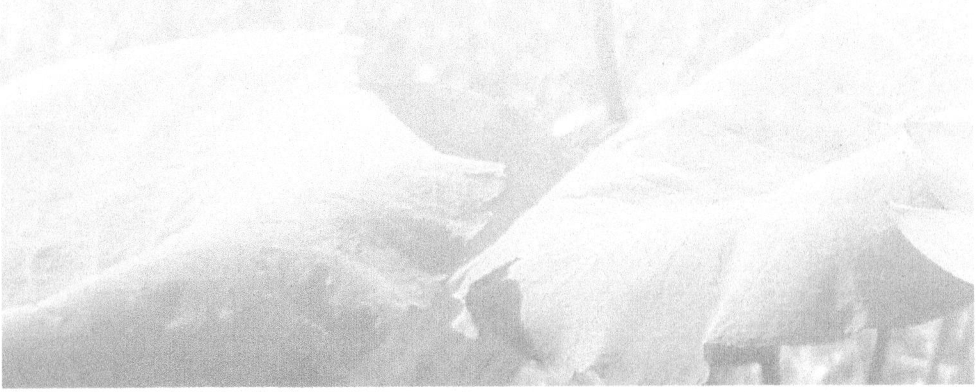

Australian Institute of Health and Welfare (2009) *Measuring the social and emotional wellbeing of Aboriginal and Torres Strait Islander Peoples.* Canberra: Australian Institute of Health and Welfare.

Australian Institute of Health and Welfare (2010) *Child Protection Australia 2008-2009.* Canberra: Australian Institute of Health and Welfare.

Beghi, M. & Rosenbaum, J.F. (2010) 'Risk factor for fatal and nonfatal repetition of suicide attempt: a critical appraisal. Current Opinion', *Psychiatry* 23:4, 349-355.

Brownhill, S., et al. (2005) 'Big build: hidden depression in men', *Australian and New Zealand Journal of Psychiatry* 39:10, 921-931.

Brunner R., et al. (2007) 'Prevalence and psychological correlates of occasional and repetitive deliberate self-harm in adolescents', *Archives of Pediatrics and Adolescent Medicine* 161:7, 641-649.

Carr-Gregg, M. (2005) *Surviving Adolescents.* Australia: Penguin Group.

Chamberlain,P., et al. (2009) 'Suicidal Ideation: The Clinical Utility of the K10', *Crisis.* 30:1, 39-42.

Connor, K. R., et al. (2003). 'Injury hospitalization and risks for subsequent self-injury and suicide: A national study from New Zealand', *American Journal of Public Health* 93:7, 1128-1131.

Corboz, J., et al. (2008) *Feeling Queer and Blue: a Review of the Literature on Depression and Related Issues among Gay, Lesbian, Bisexual and Other Homosexually Active People.* (A Report from the Australian Research Centre in Sex, Health and Society, La Trobe University, prepared for beyondblue: the national depression initiative). Melbourne: La Trobe University, Australian Research Centre in Sex, Health and Society.

De Leo, D., Sveticic, J. & Milner, A. (2011) 'Suicide in indigenous people in Queensland, Australia: trends and methods, 1994-2007', *Australian and New Zealand Journal of Psychiatry* 45:7, 532-538.

Dudgeon, Pat, et al. (2012) *Hear our Voices: Community Consultations for the Development of an Empowerment, Healing and Leadership Program for Aboriginal people living in the Kimberley, Western Australia, Final Research Report, March, 2012.* Australian Government Department of Health and Ageing

Elliott-Farrelly, T. (2004) 'Australian aboriginal suicide: the need for aboriginal suicidology?' *Australian e-Journal for the Advancement of Mental Health* 3:3, 1-8.

Farrelly, T. (2008) 'The Aboriginal Suicide and Self-Harm Help-Seeking Quandary', *Aboriginal and Islander Health Worker Journal* 32:1, January/February 2008, 11-15.

Fleischhaker, C., et al. (2011) 'Dialectical behavioral therapy for adolescents (DBT-A): a clinical trial for patients with suicidal and self-injurious behavior and borderline symptoms with a one-year follow-up', *Child and Adolescent Psychiatry and Mental Health* 5(1):3.

Goldney, R. (2002) 'Is Aboriginal Suicide Different? : A Commentary on the Work of Colin Tatz', *Psychiatry, Psychology and Law* 9(2), 257-259.

Gunnell, D., Platt, S. & Hawton, K. (2009) 'The economic crisis and suicide. Consequences may be serious and warrant early attention', *British Medical Journal* 338, 1456-1457.

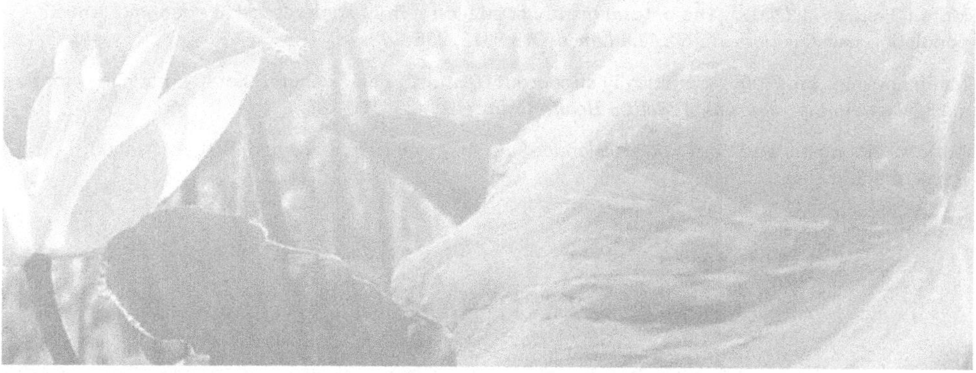

Hanssens, L. (2007) 'The search to identify contagion operating within suicide clusters in indigenous communities, Northern Territory. Australia', *Aboriginal and Islander Health Worker Journal* 31, 27-33.

Hawton, K. & Rodham, K. (2006) *By Their Own Hand: Deliberate Self Harm and Suicidal Ideas in Adolescents*. London: Jessica Kingsley Publishers.

Hillier, L., et al. (2010) *Writing Themselves in 3 (WTi3). The third national study on the sexual health and wellbeing of same sex attracted and gender questioning young people*. Melbourne: La Trobe University, Australian Research Centre in Sex, Health and Society.

Hubble, M., Duncan, B. & Miller, S. (1999) *The Heart and Soul of Change: What Works in Therapy*. Washington, DC: American Psychological Association.

In-Albon, T. (2013) 'Non-suicidal self-injury and emotion regulation: a review on facial emotion recognition and facial mimicry', *Child and Adolescent Psychiatry and Mental Health* 7:5.

Kelly, C.M. (2008) 'Development of mental health first aid guidelines for deliberate non-suicidal self-injury: A Delphi study', *BMC Psychiatry* 8:62.

Klonsky, E.D. & Muehlenkamp, J.J. (2007) 'Self-injury: A research review for the practitioner', *Journal of Clinical Psychology 63*, 1045-1056.

Koerner, K. (2012) *Doing Dialectical Behavior Theory: A Practical Guide*. New York: Guilford.

Kölves, K., Ide, N. & De Leo, D. (2011) 'Marital breakdown, shame and suicidality in men: a direct link?' *Suicide and Life-Threatening Behavior* 41:2, 149-159.

Linehan, M.M., Bohus, M. & Lynch, T. (2007) 'Dialectical behavior therapy for pervasive emotion dysregulation'. In Gross, J. (ed) *Handbook of Emotion Regulation*. New York: Guilford Press. 508-605.

Lloyd-Richardson, E.E., et al. (2007) 'Characteristics and functions of non-suicidal self-injury in a community sample of adolescents', *Psychological Medicine* 37, 1183-1192.

Madge, Nicola, et al. (2008) 'Deliberate self-harm within an international community sample of young people: comparative findings from the Child & Adolescent Self-harm in Europe' (CASE) Study', *Journal of Child Psychology and Psychiatry* 49:6, 667-677.

Martin, G. (2010) 'Self-injury in Australia: a community survey', *Medical Journal of Australia* 193:9, 506-510.

Martin, G., et al. (2010). *The Australian National Epidemiological Study of Self-Injury (ANESSI)*. Brisbane, Qld: Centre for Suicide Prevention Studies. Accessed November 23, 2012.

Menswatch Peer Support Training. See: http://aimhs.com.au/cms/index.php?page=menswatch-program

Mental Health First Aid Training and Research Program (2008). *Non-suicidal self-injury: first aid guidelines*. University of Melbourne: Orygen Youth Health Research Centre.

Miller, K. & Burns, C. (2008) 'Suicides on farms in South Australia, 1997-2001', *Australian Journal of Rural Health* 16:6, 327-331.

Moran, Paul, et al. (2012) 'The natural history of self-harm from adolescence to young adulthood: a population-based cohort study', *The Lancet* 379:9812, 236–243.

Muehlenkamp, J.L. (2006) 'Empirically supported treatments and general therapy guidelines for non-suicidal self-injury', *Journal of Mental Health Counselling* 28, 166-185.

National Aboriginal and Torres Strait Islander Suicide Prevention Strategy (2013). Australia: Department of Health.

National Action Plan for Promotion, Prevention and Early Intervention for Mental Health (2000). Mental Health and Special Programs Branch, Commonwealth Department of Health and Aged Care. Available from: http://familyconcernpublishing.com.au/wpcontent/uploads/2014/01/ActionPlanPPEi.pdf

Owens, D., Horrocks, J. & House, A. (2002) 'Fatal and non-fatal repetition of self-harm. Systematic review', *British Journal of Psychiatry* 181, 193-199.

Page, A., et al. (2007) 'Further increases in rural suicide in young Australian adults: Secular trends, 1979-2003', *Social Science and Medicine* 65:3, 442-453.

Pink, B. & Allbon, P. (2008) *The Health and Welfare of Australia's Aboriginal and Torres Strait Islander Peoples.* Commonwealth of Australia: Australian Bureau of Statistics and Australian Institute of Health and Welfare,

Pinker, S. (2002) *The Blank Slate: The Modern Denial of Human Nature.* U.S.A..Penguin.

Player, M.J., et al. (2015) 'What Interrupts Suicide Attempts in Men: a Qualitative Study', *PLoS ONE* 10:6. Available from: doi:10.1371/journal.pone.0128180

Port Lincoln Aboriginal Health Service. See: http://www.plahs.org.au/

Russell, S.T. & Toomey, R.B. (2013) 'Men's sexual orientation and suicide: evidence for US adolescent-specific risk', *Social Science & Medicine* 7:4, 523–529.

Rutz, W. & Rihmer, Z. (2009) 'Suicide in men: Suicide prevention for the male person'. In Wasserman, D. & Wasserman, C. (eds.) *Oxford textbook of suicidology and suicide prevention: a global perspective.* New York: Oxford University Press. 249-255

Sawrikar, P. (2004) *The Relationship between emotional suppression and mental health among adolescents.* Conference paper presented at 28th International Congress of Psychology, Beijing, China, 8–13 August.

Schneider, B. (2009) 'Substance use disorders and risk for completed suicide', *Archives of Suicide Research* 134, 303-316.

Schneider, B., et al. (2011) 'Impact of employment status and work-related factors on risk of completed suicide: a case-control psychological autopsy study', *Psychiatry Research* 190:2-3, 265-70. Available from: http://dx.doi.org/10.1016/j.psychres.2011.07.037

Sher, L. (2006) 'Alcohol consumption and suicide', *QJM: an international journal of medicine* 99:1, 57-61.

Skogman, K., Alsén, M. & Ojehagen, A. (2004) 'Sex differences in risk factors for suicide after attempted suicide: a follow-up study of 1052 suicide attempters', *Social Psychiatry and Psychiatric Epidemiology* 39:2, 113-120.

Steel, Z., et al. (2006) 'Pathways to the first contact with specialist mental health care', *Australian and New Zealand Journal of Psychiatry* 40:4, 347-354.

Suicide Prevention Australia (April 2008) *Suicide Prevention and Capacity Building in Australian Indigenous Communities. Position Statement.* Leichhardt, N.S.W.: Suicide Prevention Australia. Reviewed September 2010.

Suicide Prevention Australia (2009) *Suicide and self-harm among Gay, Lesbian, Bisexual and Transgender communities. Position Statement.* Leichhardt, N.S.W.: Suicide Prevention Australia.

The Elders' Report into Preventing Indigenous Self-harm & Youth Suicide (2014) Available from: https://bepartofthehealing.org/EldersReport.pdf

Wilkinson, P., et al. (2011) 'Clinical and psychosocial predictors of suicide attempts and non-suicidal self-injury in the Adolescent Depression Antidepressant and Psychotherapy Trial (ADAPT)', *American Journal of Psychiatry* 168, 495-501.

Wyder, M., Ward, P. & De Leo, D. (2009) 'Separation as a suicide risk factor', *Journal of Affective Disorders* 116, 208-213.

Yiriman Project: *Building Stories in our Young People*. See: http://www.yiriman.org.au/